# Acupressure and Food Therapy for Bradycardia

(ACU) Dr . EASWARABALA
SUBRAMANIAN
B.A.,D.C.P.,D.R.T.&A.E.,
P.G.D.B.A.,M.D.A.Y.N.,C.S.T.,
D.V.&M.S.,M.D(ACU)
AUTHOR

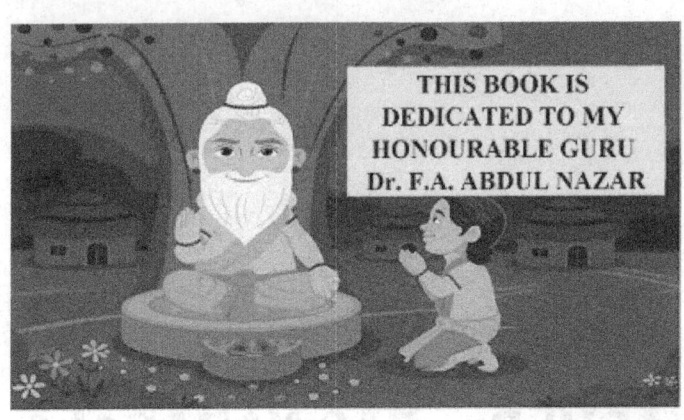

THIS BOOK IS
DEDICATED TO MY
HONOURABLE GURU
Dr. F.A. ABDUL NAZAR

# Acupressure and Food Therapy for Bradycardia

## Description

Bradycardia is a medical condition characterized by an abnormally slow heart rate. In adults, it's typically defined as a resting heart rate that falls below 60 beats per minute (bpm). However, the severity of symptoms and the need for treatment can vary depending on the individual's overall health and activity level. Bradycardia occurs when the electrical signals that regulate the heart's rhythm are disrupted, causing the heart to beat at a slower pace than normal. The heart's electrical system consists of a network of cells that generate and transmit electrical impulses, coordinating the contraction and relaxation of the heart's chambers (atria and ventricles) to pump blood effectively throughout the body.

## Causes

Bradycardia can have various causes, ranging from natural factors to medical conditions. Some common causes of bradycardia include:  Age: As people get older, their heart's electrical system can undergo natural changes that lead to a slower heart rate. This is often referred to as "age-related sinus bradycardia." Medications: Certain medications, such as beta-blockers, calcium channel blockers, and some antiarrhythmic drugs, can intentionally slow down the heart rate as a therapeutic effect. These medications are often prescribed to manage conditions like high blood pressure, heart arrhythmias, and angina.  Heart Conditions: Atrioventricular (AV) Block: This occurs when the electrical signals between the atria and ventricles are delayed or blocked, resulting in a slower heart rate. Sick Sinus Syndrome: This is a disorder where the sinus node, which generates the heart's electrical impulses, doesn't function properly, leading to episodes of bradycardia alternating with periods of rapid heart rates (tachycardia). Heart Attack: Damage to the heart's electrical system during a heart attack can disrupt normal heart rate control. Underlying Medical Conditions: Hypothyroidism: An underactive thyroid gland can lead to a decrease in the metabolic rate, including a slower heart rate. Electrolyte Imbalances: Abnormal levels of electrolytes like potassium, calcium, and magnesium can affect the heart's electrical activity and contribute to bradycardia. Hypothermia: Extremely low body temperature can slow down all bodily functions, including heart rate. Infections: Infections of the heart tissue or the surrounding areas can disrupt the heart's electrical system. Vagal Stimulation: The vagus nerve, which helps regulate various bodily functions, including heart rate, can be stimulated in ways that lead to bradycardia. For example, activities like bearing down during bowel movements or coughing forcefully can stimulate the vagus nerve and temporarily slow down the heart rate. Certain Medical Procedures: Some medical procedures, such as heart surgery, catheter ablation, or placement of a pacemaker, can directly affect the heart's electrical system and lead to temporary or permanent bradycardia. Athletic Training: Well-conditioned athletes can develop a slower resting heart rate due to their increased cardiovascular fitness. This is often referred to as "athlete's heart."  Genetic Factors: In some cases, certain genetic factors can predispose individuals to develop bradycardia.  It's important to note that the severity of bradycardia and the need for treatment depend on the individual's overall health, the presence of symptoms, and the underlying cause. If you or someone you know is experiencing symptoms of bradycardia, it's recommended to consult a healthcare professional for proper diagnosis and appropriate management.

## sign and symptoms

Bradycardia, characterized by an abnormally slow heart rate, can manifest with a variety of signs and symptoms. However, it's important to note that not everyone with bradycardia will experience noticeable symptoms. When symptoms do occur, they can vary in severity and may include: Fatigue: Individuals with bradycardia might experience excessive tiredness and a lack of energy, even with mild physical activities.  Dizziness or Lightheadedness: Reduced blood flow to the brain due to a slow heart rate can lead to feelings of dizziness or lightheadedness, especially when changing positions quickly, such as standing up from a seated or lying position. Fainting or Near-Fainting (Syncope): In some cases, bradycardia can cause a sudden drop in blood pressure, leading to episodes of fainting or almost fainting. This is particularly concerning, as it can increase the risk of falls and injuries. Shortness of Breath: Insufficient blood flow caused by a slow heart rate may lead to inadequate oxygen supply to the body's tissues, resulting in feelings of breathlessness even during mild exertion. Chest Discomfort: Some individuals may experience chest pain, discomfort, or a sensation of pressure. This can be due to reduced blood flow to the heart muscle. Palpitations:

Paradoxically, some people with bradycardia might experience a sensation of irregular or skipped heartbeats (palpitations) as the heart tries to compensate for the slower rhythm.  Confusion or Difficulty Concentrating: Inadequate blood flow to the brain can lead to cognitive symptoms such as confusion, difficulty concentrating, or memory problems.  Cool and Pale Skin: Reduced blood circulation might result in cooler or paler skin, especially in the extremities.  Weakness: A slower heart rate can lead to reduced blood supply to muscles and tissues, causing weakness and reduced physical endurance.  Exercise Intolerance: Individuals with bradycardia may find it challenging to engage in physical activities or exercises that they used to handle comfortably due to inadequate cardiac output. It's important to remember that the severity and presence of symptoms can vary based on factors such as the underlying cause of bradycardia, an individual's overall health, and their level of physical activity. Some individuals, especially athletes, may have a naturally low resting heart rate without experiencing symptoms. If you or someone else is experiencing severe symptoms like fainting, chest pain, or significant shortness of breath, seek immediate medical attention. Even if symptoms are milder, if you suspect you might have bradycardia or are experiencing concerning symptoms, it's advisable to consult a healthcare professional for proper evaluation and diagnosis.

## Organs

Bradycardia, or an abnormally slow heart rate, can affect various organs and systems in the body due to the reduced pumping efficiency of the heart. The slower heart rate leads to a decreased cardiac output, which can impact blood flow and oxygen supply to different tissues and organs. Here are some of the organs that can be affected due to bradycardia:  Brain: Insufficient blood flow to the brain can result in symptoms such as dizziness, lightheadedness, confusion, difficulty concentrating, and in severe cases, fainting (syncope). Prolonged inadequate blood supply to the brain can lead to cognitive impairment and even unconsciousness.  Heart: While it might seem counterintuitive, bradycardia itself can affect the heart. If the heart rate is too slow, it might not be able to pump an adequate amount of blood to meet the body's needs, which can strain the heart and potentially lead to heart failure over time. Kidneys: Reduced blood flow to the kidneys can affect their ability to filter waste products and maintain proper electrolyte balance, potentially leading to kidney dysfunction. Lungs: Inadequate cardiac output can lead to reduced blood flow to the lungs, affecting the exchange of oxygen and carbon dioxide. This can contribute to shortness of breath and exercise intolerance.  Muscles and Extremities: Decreased blood flow to muscles and extremities can result in weakness, fatigue, and cold or pale skin.  Digestive System: Inadequate blood supply to the digestive organs can lead to issues such as nausea, vomiting, and abdominal discomfort. Digestion may also be impaired.  Skin: Poor circulation can result in cool, pale skin due to reduced blood flow to the peripheral blood vessels.  Exercise Tolerance: Bradycardia can limit an individual's ability to engage in physical activities due to reduced cardiac output. This can impact overall physical fitness and endurance. Endocrine System: The endocrine system, which includes hormone-secreting glands like the thyroid, can be affected by bradycardia due to reduced blood flow and oxygen supply. This can impact metabolism and hormonal regulation.  Immune System: Prolonged periods of reduced blood flow can potentially weaken the immune response, making the body more susceptible to infections.  It's important to note that the extent to which these organs are affected can vary depending on factors such as the severity of the bradycardia, the individual's overall health, and the presence of underlying medical conditions. If you suspect you have bradycardia or are experiencing symptoms related to an abnormal heart rate, seeking medical attention is important for proper evaluation, diagnosis, and appropriate management.

## Age group

Bradycardia, or an abnormally slow heart rate, can affect individuals of all age groups, from infants to the elderly. However, the prevalence and causes of bradycardia can vary across different age ranges.

Here's how bradycardia can affect different age groups: Infants and Children: Bradycardia can be more concerning in infants and children, as their hearts naturally beat faster than in adults. In this age group, bradycardia is often associated with congenital heart defects, problems with the heart's electrical system, or other underlying medical conditions. It may require prompt medical attention and intervention. Adolescents and Young Adults: While bradycardia is less common in this age group, it can still occur. Athletes, in particular, might have a lower resting heart rate due to their high level of cardiovascular fitness. However, if there are associated symptoms or the heart rate drops to levels that are too low, medical evaluation is recommended.  Adults: Bradycardia can affect adults of all ages. Common causes include age-related changes in the heart's electrical system, heart conditions such as atrioventricular (AV) block, sick sinus syndrome, and the use of certain medications. Adults with other medical conditions, such as hypothyroidism or electrolyte imbalances, can also develop bradycardia. Elderly: Bradycardia becomes more prevalent as people age. Natural changes in the heart's electrical system and the degeneration of the conduction system can lead to a slower heart rate. Elderly individuals are also more likely to have underlying heart conditions that can contribute to bradycardia. Athletes: Well-conditioned athletes, regardless of age, can experience bradycardia due to their high level of physical fitness. This is often termed "athlete's heart." In athletes, bradycardia is generally considered a physiological response to their cardiovascular training rather than a pathological condition. It's important to note that while bradycardia can occur in any age group, the impact and severity of symptoms, as well as the need for treatment, can vary. In some cases, bradycardia might not cause noticeable symptoms and may not require treatment. However, if you suspect you or someone else has bradycardia or is experiencing symptoms related to an abnormal heart rate, it's advisable to seek medical evaluation to determine the underlying cause and appropriate management.

## Climatic Condition

Climatic conditions, particularly extreme temperatures, can have an impact on heart rate and potentially contribute to the development or exacerbation of bradycardia in susceptible individuals. Here's how different climatic conditions might affect bradycardia: Cold Weather: Cold weather can stimulate the body's "fight or flight" response, leading to an increase in heart rate and blood pressure. However, in individuals with preexisting heart conditions or those who are particularly sensitive to cold temperatures, the body's response to cold might be different. Cold temperatures can lead to vasoconstriction (narrowing of blood vessels), which might affect blood flow to the heart and other organs. This can potentially contribute to bradycardia, especially in individuals with compromised cardiovascular systems. Hot Weather: In hot weather, the body often tries to cool down by increasing blood flow to the skin's surface and by dilating blood vessels. This can lead to a decrease in blood pressure and heart rate as the body redistributes blood to help dissipate heat. In some cases, particularly in individuals who are not well-hydrated or have certain medical conditions, the drop in blood pressure and heart rate due to heat exposure can exacerbate or trigger bradycardia.  Extreme Environments: Extreme environments, such as high altitudes, can also impact heart rate. At high altitudes, where oxygen levels are lower, the body might respond with an increased heart rate to compensate for decreased oxygen delivery. However, in individuals who are not acclimatized to high altitudes or who have existing cardiovascular conditions, this response might be impaired, potentially leading to bradycardia.  It's important to note that while climatic conditions can influence heart rate, they are more likely to affect individuals who are already predisposed to bradycardia due to underlying medical conditions, age, fitness level, or genetic factors. Additionally, the effects of climate on heart rate can vary from person to person.  If you have concerns about how climatic conditions might be affecting your heart rate or if you have a history of heart conditions, it's a good idea to take necessary precautions, such as staying hydrated, avoiding extreme temperature changes, and consulting a healthcare professional for guidance on managing your heart health in different environments.

## Region

Bradycardia, as a medical condition, can affect individuals worldwide, regardless of geographic regions. The prevalence and causes of bradycardia can be influenced by factors such as genetics, lifestyle, healthcare access, and environmental conditions. Here's how different regions worldwide can be affected by bradycardia:  Developed Countries: In developed countries with advanced healthcare systems, individuals with bradycardia have better access to medical diagnosis and treatment. However, the prevalence of bradycardia can still vary based on factors such as aging populations, lifestyle choices, and the presence of risk factors for heart conditions. Developing Countries: In some developing countries, access to healthcare resources might be more limited, leading to underdiagnosis or undertreatment of bradycardia. Factors such as inadequate medical facilities, lack of awareness, and economic challenges can contribute to variations in the recognition and management of bradycardia. Urban vs. Rural Areas: There might be differences in the prevalence and management of bradycardia between urban and rural areas. Urban populations might have better access to medical care and diagnostic tools, while rural populations could face challenges in accessing healthcare services, leading to disparities in diagnosis and treatment.  Climate and Altitude: Certain geographic regions with extreme climates, high altitudes, or harsh environmental conditions might have a higher incidence of bradycardia due to the effects of climate and oxygen availability on heart rate regulation. Individuals living in such regions might experience adaptations in their heart rates to better cope with the local conditions.  Genetic and Ethnic Factors: Genetic factors play a significant role in heart health, and different ethnic groups may have varying predispositions to heart conditions, including bradycardia. Certain genetic traits and variations can influence how the heart's electrical system functions, contributing to differences in the prevalence of bradycardia across populations.  Lifestyle and Dietary Habits: Cultural differences in lifestyle, physical activity, and dietary habits can impact the overall heart health of populations. Unhealthy lifestyle choices, such as high-fat diets, smoking, excessive alcohol consumption, and lack of physical activity, can increase the risk of heart conditions, including bradycardia.  It's important to note that while bradycardia can affect people worldwide, its prevalence, causes, and impact can vary based on the factors mentioned above. Regardless of geographic region, individuals who experience symptoms of bradycardia or have concerns about their heart health should seek medical evaluation and guidance from healthcare professionals.

## LAB TEST

Diagnosing the underlying cause of bradycardia typically involves a combination of medical history assessment, physical examination, and various laboratory tests. The specific tests conducted will depend on the suspected cause of the bradycardia, the presence of symptoms, and the individual's medical history. Here are some common laboratory tests that might be used to diagnose bradycardia: Electrocardiogram (ECG or EKG): An ECG is a fundamental test used to diagnose bradycardia. It records the electrical activity of the heart and can identify abnormalities in heart rate and rhythm. A prolonged PR interval or an irregular rhythm on the ECG might indicate underlying heart conduction problems. Holter Monitor: A Holter monitor is a portable device that records the heart's electrical activity continuously over 24 to 48 hours. It provides a more extended period of monitoring than a standard ECG and can capture episodes of bradycardia that might not occur during a short ECG.  Event Monitor: Similar to a Holter monitor, an event monitor is used for longer-term monitoring. It's typically worn for a few weeks or until an episode of bradycardia occurs. When the individual experiences symptoms, they can activate the monitor to record the heart's activity during that time.  Blood Tests: Blood tests might be performed to check for underlying medical conditions that can contribute to bradycardia. For example: Thyroid function tests: To assess thyroid hormone levels, as hypothyroidism can cause bradycardia. Electrolyte levels: Imbalances in electrolytes like potassium and calcium can affect heart rhythm. Cardiac enzyme levels: To check for damage to heart tissue, which can sometimes be related to bradycardia. Exercise Stress Test: This test involves monitoring the heart's response to exercise. It can help reveal abnormal heart rhythms or a drop in heart rate during physical activity. Tilt Table Test: This test is used to evaluate the body's response to changes in position. It can help diagnose conditions that cause bradycardia or fainting upon standing up. Electrophysiological Studies (EPS): EPS involves inserting catheters into the heart to study its electrical activity. It's typically performed in more complex cases of bradycardia to locate the precise location of the conduction problems. Genetic Testing: In some cases, genetic testing might be considered, especially if there's a family history of inherited heart conditions that could cause bradycardia. Remember that the choice of tests will depend on the clinical judgment of the healthcare professional. If you suspect you have bradycardia or are experiencing symptoms related to an abnormal heart rate, it's important to consult a healthcare provider. They will determine which tests are most appropriate based on your individual circumstances.

## Best Diet

Maintaining a healthy diet is important for overall heart health, and it can be beneficial for individuals with bradycardia as well. While there's no specific diet that directly targets bradycardia, adopting a heart-healthy eating pattern can support your cardiovascular system and overall well-being. Here are some dietary guidelines that might be beneficial for individuals with bradycardia: Eat a Balanced Diet: Consume a variety of nutrient-rich foods to ensure you're getting a well-rounded mix of vitamins, minerals, fiber, and antioxidants. Focus on whole foods like fruits, vegetables, whole grains, lean proteins, and healthy fats.  Limit Saturated and Trans Fats: Minimize your intake of saturated and trans fats, as these can contribute to heart disease. Choose sources of healthy fats, such as avocados, nuts, seeds, and fatty fish like salmon.  Choose Lean Proteins: Opt for lean protein sources like poultry, fish, legumes, beans, and tofu. Limit processed and red meats, which can be high in saturated fats.  Incorporate Fruits and Vegetables: Aim to fill half your plate with colorful fruits and vegetables. They are rich in vitamins, minerals, and antioxidants that support heart health.  Whole Grains: Choose whole grains like brown rice, quinoa, whole wheat bread, and whole grain pasta instead of refined grains. They provide more fiber and nutrients. Healthy Fluid Intake: Staying well-hydrated is important for heart health. Aim for water as your primary beverage and limit sugary drinks and excessive caffeine, as they might affect heart rhythm. Limit Sodium Intake: Excessive sodium can lead to high blood pressure, which can impact heart health. Reduce your sodium intake by minimizing processed and packaged foods and using herbs and spices for flavoring.  Omega-3 Fatty Acids: Include sources of omega-3 fatty acids, such as fatty fish (salmon, mackerel, sardines), flaxseeds, chia seeds, and walnuts. Omega-3s have been associated with heart health.  Monitor Caffeine Intake: While moderate caffeine consumption is generally safe for most people, some individuals might be more sensitive to its effects on heart rate. Monitor your caffeine intake and its impact on your heart rate.  Stay Hydrated: Proper hydration is essential for heart health. Dehydration can potentially impact heart rhythm, so ensure you're drinking enough water throughout the day. Limit Alcohol: If you consume alcohol, do so in moderation. Excessive alcohol intake can have negative effects on the heart.  Customize to Individual Needs: Everyone's dietary needs are unique. If you have specific dietary restrictions, medical conditions, or concerns, consult a healthcare professional or registered dietitian for personalized guidance.  Remember, adopting a healthy lifestyle that includes regular physical activity, maintaining a healthy weight, managing stress, and getting adequate sleep are all crucial components of supporting your heart health, especially if you have bradycardia or other heart-related concerns. Always consult a healthcare professional before making significant changes to your diet or lifestyle.

## Vegetables Diet

A diet rich in vegetables can be highly beneficial for individuals with bradycardia and anyone looking to support their heart health. Vegetables are low in calories, high in fiber, and packed with vitamins, minerals, and antioxidants that contribute to overall well-being and cardiovascular health. Here's a list of vegetables you might consider including in your diet: Leafy Greens:  Spinach Kale Swiss chard Collard greens Romaine lettuce Cruciferous Vegetables:  Broccoli Cauliflower Brussels sprouts

Cabbage Colorful Vegetables: Bell peppers (red, yellow, orange) Carrots Tomatoes Sweet potatoes Root Vegetables: Beets Radishes Turnips Carrots Allium Vegetables: Garlic Onions Leeks Legumes: Beans (black beans, kidney beans, pinto beans) Lentils Chickpeas Peas: Green peas Snow peas Snap peas Zucchini and Squash: Zucchini Yellow squash Butternut squash Cucumbers: Cucumbers Mushrooms: Various types of mushrooms Including a variety of these vegetables in your diet can provide numerous health benefits. Here are some reasons why vegetables are important for individuals with bradycardia: Rich in

Antioxidants: Vegetables are high in antioxidants that help protect cells from damage caused by free radicals, which can contribute to heart disease and other chronic conditions. High in Fiber: Fiber supports digestive health and helps regulate blood sugar levels. It can also help manage cholesterol levels, which is important for heart health. Low in Saturated Fat: Most vegetables are naturally low in saturated fat, making them a heart-healthy choice. Rich in Potassium: Potassium is an essential mineral that plays a role in maintaining a healthy heart rhythm. Many vegetables, such as leafy greens, tomatoes, and potatoes, are good sources of

potassium.  Blood Pressure
Regulation: Certain vegetables
contain compounds that may
help regulate blood pressure,
which is important for overall
cardiovascular health.  Weight
Management: A diet rich in
vegetables can contribute to
weight management, which is
beneficial for heart health,
especially for individuals with
bradycardia.  Remember to
prepare vegetables in ways
that retain their nutritional
value, such as steaming,
roasting, or lightly sautéing.
Aim to include a variety of
colors and types of vegetables
to ensure you're getting a
diverse range of nutrients. If
you have specific dietary
restrictions or health concerns,
consider consulting a

registered dietitian for personalized guidance.

## Fruits Diet

Incorporating a variety of fruits into your diet can provide essential nutrients, fiber, and antioxidants that support overall health, including heart health for individuals with bradycardia. Fruits are naturally low in calories, rich in vitamins, minerals, and phytochemicals, and they can contribute to a well-rounded and balanced diet. Here are some fruits to consider including in your diet:  Berries: Blueberries Strawberries Raspberries Blackberries Citrus Fruits:  Oranges Grapefruits Lemons Limes Apples and Pears:  Apples Pears Bananas:

Bananas Tropical Fruits: Pineapples Mangos Papayas Kiwi Stone Fruits:  Peaches Plums Cherries Melons: Watermelon Cantaloupe Honeydew Grapes:  Red grapes Green grapes Avocado: Avocado (technically a fruit) Here are some reasons why incorporating fruits into your diet can be beneficial for individuals with bradycardia: Rich in Vitamins and Minerals: Fruits provide essential vitamins and minerals that support overall health, including cardiovascular health.  Antioxidant Content: Fruits are high in antioxidants, which help protect cells from oxidative stress and inflammation that can contribute to heart disease.

Fiber: Many fruits are a good source of dietary fiber, which supports digestive health, helps manage blood sugar levels, and can help control cholesterol levels.  Potassium: Some fruits, such as bananas, oranges, and cantaloupe, are rich in potassium, an electrolyte that plays a role in maintaining a healthy heart rhythm.  Hydration: Fruits have high water content, contributing to hydration, which is important for maintaining optimal heart function.  Natural Sweetness: Fruits can satisfy your sweet cravings without relying on added sugars, which can be harmful to heart health.  When incorporating fruits into your diet, aim for a variety of colors to ensure you're getting a diverse range of nutrients. Fresh, frozen, and canned fruits (in natural juice or water) can all be good choices. If you have specific dietary restrictions or health concerns, consulting a registered dietitian can help you create a personalized plan that suits your needs and supports your heart health.

## Acupuncture is a most efficient is an alternative treatment

### What is Acupuncture?
It is an interesting perspective to consider that Acupuncture

and its Five Element theory originated in India and spread to other parts of the world through Buddhism. The influence of Buddhism in the spread of Acupuncture in countries like China, Japan, Korea, Indonesia, Taiwan, Vietnam, Hong Kong, and Sri Lanka is indeed noteworthy. The Vedas, ancient texts from India, have mentioned Acupuncture as an art of healing and an anaesthetic tool during surgical procedures about 7000 years ago, which highlights the rich history of Acupuncture in India. However, for various reasons, Buddhism did not flourish in India, and Acupuncture did not gain popularity in the region.

Instead, the path of self-discovery in India transformed into Yoga, which later gave birth to Acupuncture as a means of maintaining the vital energy in health and disease. Yoga requires devotion, dedication, discipline, and practice under the guidance of a guru, and it can be challenging. Therefore, the system of Srotan, Nadi, and Murma, which is synonymous with Acupuncture meridians and points, was developed in India so that experts could assess the harmony of the body through Nadi Vigyan or pulse diagnosis.

This historical perspective sheds light on the interconnectedness of different healing practices and how they have evolved and spread across different regions of the world. It also emphasizes the significance of cultural influences in the development and popularity of certain healing modalities in specific regions.

Acupuncture is often used to treat a wide range of conditions, including pain, allergies, depression, anxiety, insomnia, digestive disorders, and infertility. It is often used in conjunction with other forms of traditional Chinese medicine, such as herbal medicine and cupping therapy. The needles used in acupuncture are very thin, and the insertion process is generally painless. The acupuncturist will insert the needles into specific points on the body, depending on the patient's symptoms and the condition being treated. Once the needles are in place, they may be manipulated by the acupuncturist, using techniques such as gentle twisting or tapping, to enhance the treatment's effectiveness.

Acupuncture is generally considered safe when performed by a trained and licensed practitioner. However, there are some risks associated with the practice, including bleeding, infection, and organ puncture. Patients should always make sure to seek treatment from a qualified practitioner and discuss any potential risks or side effects with their healthcare provider.

In conclusion, acupuncture is a form of alternative medicine that involves the insertion of thin needles into specific points on the body to stimulate the body's natural healing process and restore the flow of Qi. It is used to treat a wide range of conditions and is generally considered safe when performed by a trained and licensed practitioner.

## Types of Acupuncture

There are several types of acupuncture practiced around the world. Here are some of the most common types:

Acupuncture and its Five Element theory originated in India and spread to other parts of the world through Buddhism. The influence of Buddhism in the spread of Acupuncture in countries like China, Japan, Korea, Indonesia, Taiwan, Vietnam, Hong Kong, and Sri Lanka is indeed noteworthy.

Traditional Chinese acupuncture: This is the most common form of acupuncture and is based on the traditional principles of Chinese medicine. It involves inserting needles into specific points along the meridians to balance the flow of Qi.
Japanese acupuncture: This form of acupuncture is similar

to traditional Chinese acupuncture but uses thinner needles and shallower insertion. It also focuses more on palpation and diagnosis of the meridians and points.

Korean acupuncture: This form of acupuncture is similar to Chinese acupuncture but places more emphasis on the hands and feet. It also uses more needle stimulation techniques, such as heat, electricity, or herbs.

Ear acupuncture: Also known as auricular acupuncture, this form of acupuncture involves inserting needles into specific points on the ear. It is often used to treat addiction, pain, and mental health conditions.

Scalp acupuncture: This form of acupuncture involves inserting needles into specific points on the scalp. It is often used to treat neurological conditions such as stroke or Parkinson's disease.

Trigger point acupuncture: This form of acupuncture focuses on specific points of muscle tension or "trigger points" and uses needles to release the tension and relieve pain.

Electroacupuncture: This form of acupuncture involves attaching electrodes to the needles and sending a small electrical current through them. It is often used to treat

pain and nerve-related
conditions.

Each type of acupuncture has
its own unique approach and
techniques, and a trained
acupuncturist will choose the
best type for the patient's
needs and condition.

## Acupuncture Needles

Acupuncture needles are thin,
sterile, and disposable needles
made of stainless steel, silver,
or gold. They come in different
lengths, widths, and gauges
(thickness). The length of the
needle can range from 0.5 inch
to several inches, depending
on the area being treated. The
width and gauge can also vary,
with thinner needles used for
more delicate areas, such as

the face or ears, and thicker needles used for larger muscle groups.

Acupuncture needles are designed to be very thin and flexible, so they can be inserted into the skin with minimal discomfort. They are typically single-use needles that are disposed of after each treatment to prevent infection and ensure safety. Most needles are made with a guide tube or insertion tube that helps to guide the needle into the skin and minimize discomfort.

The needles are inserted into specific points along the meridians or energy pathways of the body. The acupuncturist will determine the appropriate depth and angle of insertion based on the patient's condition and the area being treated. Once the needles are in place, they may be gently manipulated by the acupuncturist to enhance the treatment's effectiveness.

Acupuncture needles are generally considered safe when used by a trained and licensed practitioner. However, there are some risks associated with the practice, such as infection or organ puncture, so it's important to seek treatment from a qualified practitioner and discuss any potential risks or side effects with your healthcare provider.

# Needle

Acupuncture needles are typically made of stainless steel, silver, or gold. Here's a brief overview of each type of material:

Stainless steel: Stainless steel needles are the most common type of acupuncture needles used today. They are made of medical-grade stainless steel, which is durable, rust-resistant, and easy to sterilize. Stainless steel needles are relatively affordable, and they come in various lengths, widths, and gauges to accommodate different treatment needs.

Silver: Silver needles are less commonly used than stainless steel needles and are considered to be more expensive. They are typically made of pure silver or silver-plated brass. Silver is believed to have certain therapeutic properties according to traditional Chinese medicine, such as being able to enhance the flow of Qi and blood. Silver needles are often used for specific conditions or for patients who are more sensitive to other metals.

Gold: Gold needles are the least commonly used type of acupuncture needles due to their high cost. They are typically made of pure gold or gold-plated brass. Gold is believed to have certain properties, such as being able to tonify Qi and calm the mind, according to traditional Chinese medicine. Gold needles are often used for specific conditions or for patients with certain sensitivities.

It's worth noting that the material of the acupuncture needle itself does not necessarily determine the effectiveness of the treatment. The therapeutic effects of acupuncture are primarily based on the skill and expertise of the acupuncturist, the location of the needle insertion, and the patient's individual response to the treatment. The choice of needle material may be based on personal preferences or specific treatment protocols followed by the acupuncturist.

## Regions

Acupuncture has been widely practiced in various regions of the world for centuries. Here are some of the regions where acupuncture has been historically accepted and widely used:

The Vedas, ancient texts from India, have mentioned Acupuncture as an art of healing and an anaesthetic tool during surgical procedures about 7000 years ago, which highlights the rich history of Acupuncture in India. However, for various reasons, Buddhism did not flourish in India, and

Acupuncture did not gain popularity in the region.

China: Acupuncture originated in China over 2,000 years ago and has been a part of Chinese medicine ever since. Acupuncture is still widely practiced in China today, both in traditional and modern medical settings.

Japan: Acupuncture was introduced to Japan in the 6th century, and Japanese acupuncture has its own unique techniques and styles. It is still widely practiced in Japan today.

Korea: Acupuncture has been practiced in Korea for over 1,500 years, and Korean acupuncture has its own unique techniques and styles. It is still widely practiced in Korea today, and is often combined with other traditional Korean medicine practices.

Southeast Asia: Acupuncture has been practiced in Southeast Asia for centuries, particularly in countries like Vietnam, Thailand, and Indonesia. It is often combined with other traditional healing practices, such as herbal medicine and massage.

Europe: Acupuncture was introduced to Europe in the 16th century by Jesuit missionaries and has since become increasingly popular. It is now widely practiced in many European countries, particularly in France, Germany, and the UK.

North America: Acupuncture was introduced to North America in the 19th century and has since become increasingly popular. It is now widely practiced in the United States and Canada, both in traditional and modern medical settings.

Latin America: Acupuncture has been practiced in Latin America for

several decades, particularly in countries like Brazil and Argentina. It is often used in combination with other traditional healing practices.

Acupuncture is considered a safe and effective form of complementary and alternative medicine, and its popularity continues to grow worldwide.

## Acupuncture and Acupressure

## Technique

Acupuncture involves the insertion of thin needles into specific points on the body, known as acupoints or acupuncture points. These needles are typically manipulated by hand or through electrical stimulation to achieve the desired effect. Acupressure, on the other hand, utilizes pressure applied to the same acupoints using fingers, palms, elbows, or specialized tools. No needles are involved in acupressure.

## Stimulation

Acupuncture stimulates the acupoints by inserting needles, which are believed to help restore the flow of energy (qi) along the body's meridians. Acupressure stimulates the acupoints through pressure, aiming to unblock any energy stagnation and restore balance in the body.

# Sensation

During acupuncture, patients may feel sensations such as tingling, warmth, or a dull ache at the site of needle insertion. These sensations are often considered part of the therapeutic process. Acupressure typically produces sensations of pressure and sometimes discomfort, but it does not involve the unique sensations associated with needle insertion.

## Application

Acupuncture is typically performed by trained acupuncturists who insert needles at precise depths and angles based on the patient's condition and traditional Chinese medicine principles. Acupressure can be self-administered or performed by others, and it is relatively easy to learn basic techniques for self-care.

## Duration

Acupuncture sessions usually last around 20 to 30 minutes, with the patient lying still while the needles are in place. Acupressure sessions can vary in duration depending on the techniques used and the specific condition being treated. They may be shorter or longer than acupuncture sessions.

## Safety Considerations

Acupuncture should be performed by trained and licensed practitioners to minimize the risk of complications such as infection or injury from needle insertion. Acupressure is generally considered safe for most people when performed correctly, but it may not be suitable for individuals with certain medical conditions or during pregnancy.

Both acupuncture and acupressure are based on the principles of traditional Indian medicine and aim to promote health and well-being by restoring the body's natural balance. However, they differ in their techniques, application, and sensations experienced by the patient.

Apply pressure in a circular motion using your single finger on the following points for 30 seconds to 2 minutes.

By following the these recommendations, one can improve their lifestyle. The time duration for seeing improvements may differ from person to person.

# I will give below acupuncture points.

## ST 36

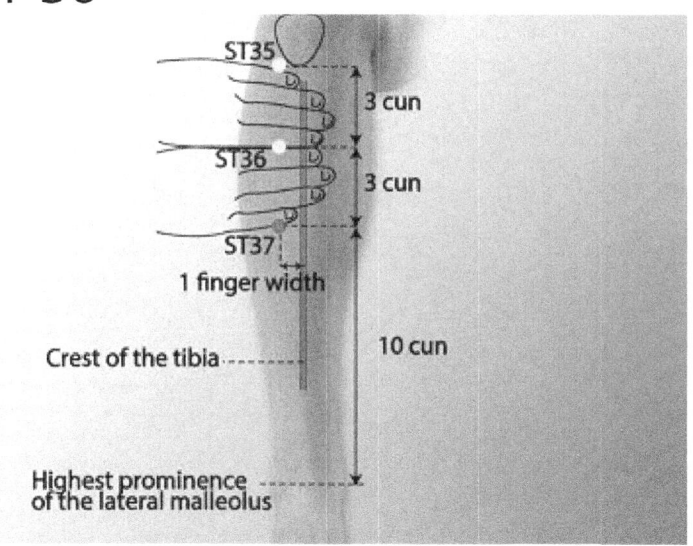

SP 6

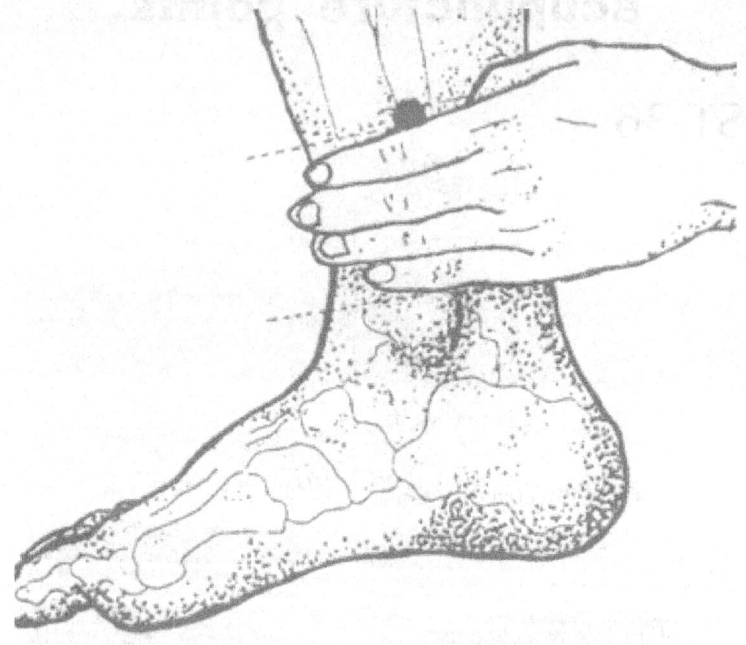

# H 7

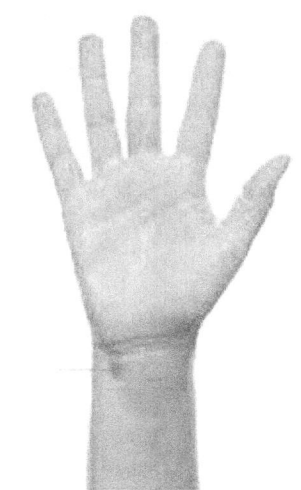

# PC 6

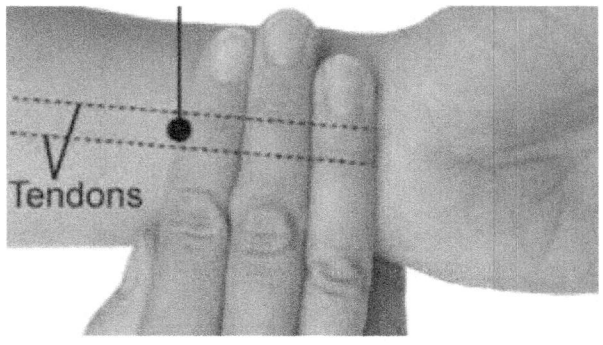

Tendons

# CV 14

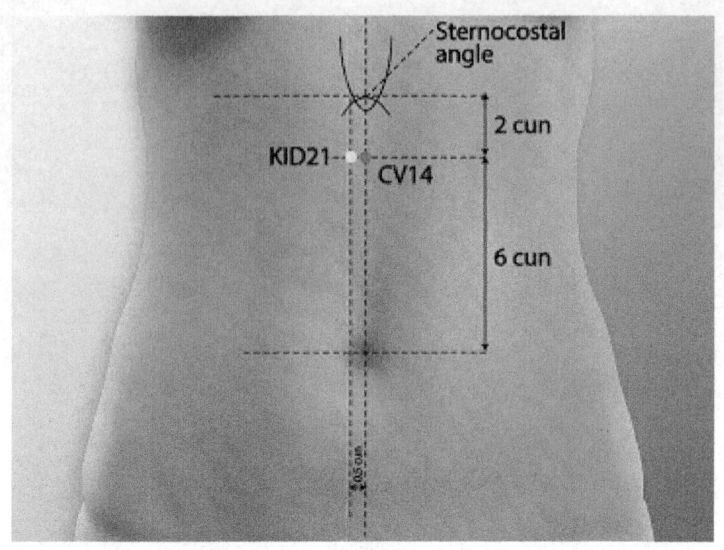

# BL 15

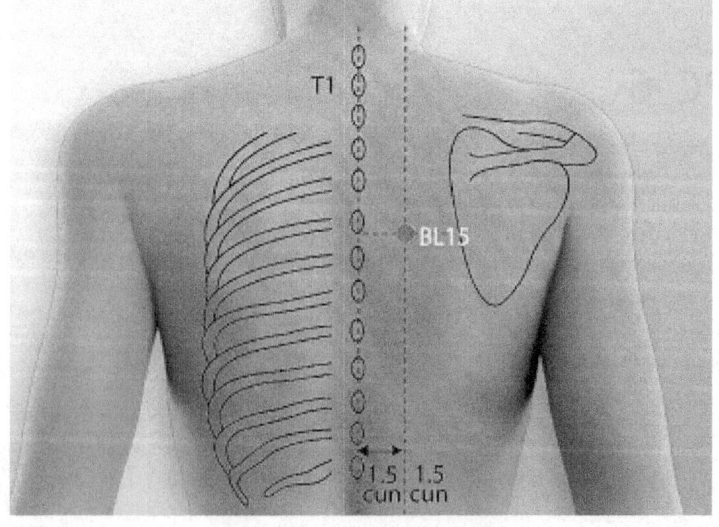

# EXHN 3

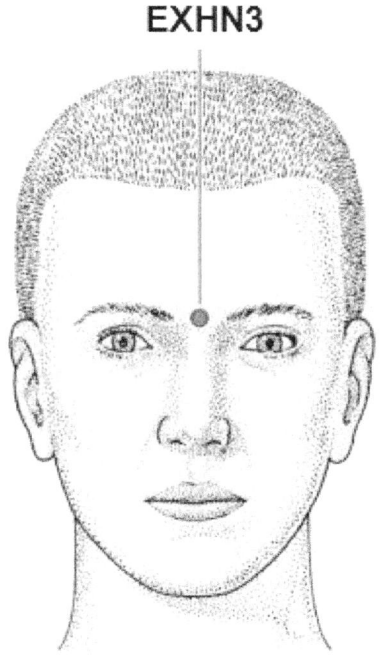

EXHN3

# LI 4

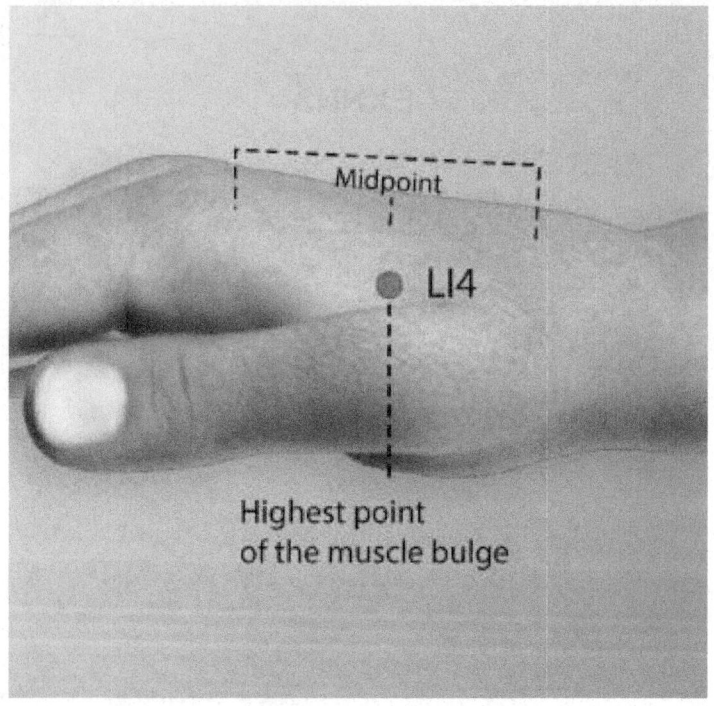

Midpoint

LI4

Highest point
of the muscle bulge

# LU 9

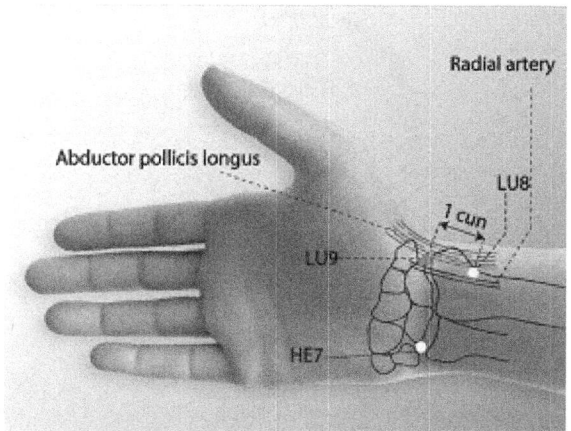

# LI 10

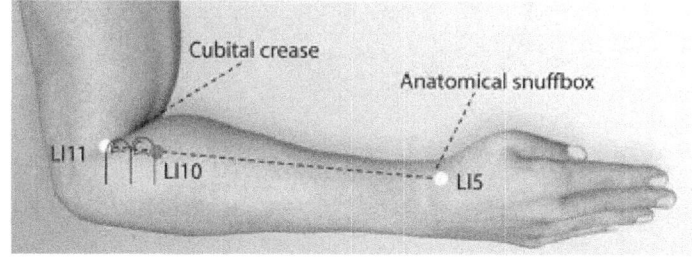

# GV 20

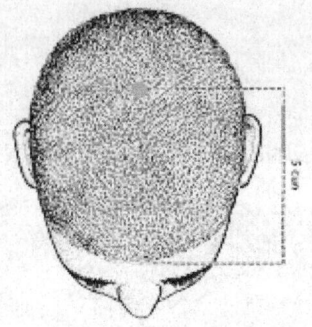

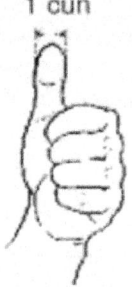
1 cun

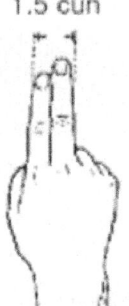
1.5 cun

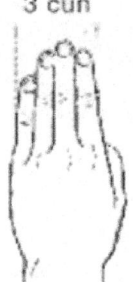
3 cun

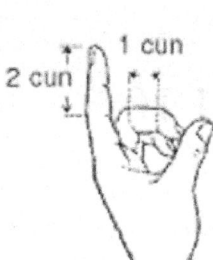
2 cun   1 cun

# OTHER BOOKS

| | |
|---|---|
| | Chickenpox |
| 28 | (varicella) |
| 29 | Chikungunya |
| 30 | Chlamydia |
| 31 | Cholera |
| 32 | Chronic Fatigue Syndrome |
| 33 | Chronic Obstructive Pulmonary Disease (COPD) |
| 34 | Ciguatera fish poisoning (CFP) |
| 35 | Clostridium difficile infection |
| 36 | Congenital heart disease |
| 37 | Congenital rubella |
| 38 | Congenital syphilis |
| 39 | Conjunctivitis |

| | |
|---|---|
| 40 | Cowpox |
| 41 | Coxsackie virus |
| 42 | Crabs |
| 43 | Creutzfeldt-Jakob disease |
| 44 | Crimean-Congo haemorrhagic fever |
| 45 | Cryptosporidiosis |
| 46 | Cutaneous warts |
| 47 | Cyclospora |
| 48 | Dengue |
| 49 | Diphtheria |
| 50 | E. Coli |
| 51 | Eastern Equine Encephalitis Virus (EEEV) |
| 52 | Ebola haemorrhagic fever |
| 53 | Echinococcosis |
| 54 | Ehrlichiosis |

| | |
|---|---|
| 68 | Giardiasis |
| 69 | Gout |
| 70 | Group A Gonorrhoea |
| 71 | Group A Streptococcus |
| 72 | Haemophilus infection |
| 73 | Haemorrhagic |
| 74 | Haemorrhagic fever |
| 75 | Haff Disease |
| 76 | Hantavirus infection |
| 77 | Harmful Algal Blooms |
| 78 | Head Lice |
| 79 | Heart failure |
| 80 | Heat-related Illnesses |
| 81 | Helicobacter Pylori |
| 82 | Hepatitis |
| 83 | Hepatitis A |

| | |
|---|---|
| 84 | Hepatitis B |
| 85 | Hepatitis C |
| 86 | Hepatitis E |
| 87 | High Blood Pressure |
| 88 | Histoplasmosis |
| 89 | Human Metapneumovirus |
| 90 | Human papillomavirus infection (HPV) |
| 91 | Hydatidosis |
| 92 | Hypertensive heart disease |
| 93 | Incontinence |
| 94 | Inflammatory cardiomegaly |
| 95 | Influenza A (H9N2) |
| 96 | Invasive meningococcal disease |

disease

# Vaginitis

# Part 2

## Part 3

Appendicitis

Body Lice

# Chronic Hepatitis

| | |
|---|---|
| 570 | Irritable Bowel Syndrome (IBS) |
| 571 | Jock Itch (Tinea Cruris) |
| 572 | Kawasaki Syndrome |
| 573 | Keratitis |
| 574 | Kidney Failure |
| 575 | Knee Sprain |
| 576 | Lacunar Stroke |
| 577 | Laryngitis |
| 578 | Lazy Eye (Amblyopia) |
| 579 | Leg Strain |
| 580 | Liver Cancer |
| 581 | Lung Cancer |
| 582 | Lymphoma |
| 583 | Major Depression |
| 584 | Malignant Hyperthermia |
| 585 | Maturity Onset Diabetes of the Young (MODY) |

Made in the USA
Las Vegas, NV
16 October 2024

96943457R00075